48 Sore Throat Juicing Solutions:

Strengthen Your Immune System with These Life Changing Juice Recipes and Cure Your Sore Throat

By

Joe Correa CSN

COPYRIGHT

ACKNOWLEDGEMENTS

This book is dedicated to my friends and family that have had mild or serious illnesses so that you may find a solution and make the necessary changes in your life.

48 Sore Throat Juicing Solutions:

Strengthen Your Immune System with These Life Changing Juice Recipes and Cure Your Sore Throat

By

Joe Correa CSN

CONTENTS

Copyright

Acknowledgements

About The Author

Introduction

Commitment

48 Sore Throat Juicing Solutions: Strengthen Your Immune System with These Life Changing Juice Recipes and Cure Your Sore Throat

Additional Titles from This Author

ABOUT THE AUTHOR

After years of Research, I honestly believe in the positive effects that proper nutrition can have over the body and mind. My knowledge and experience has helped me live healthier throughout the years and which I have shared with family and friends. The more you know about eating and drinking healthier, the sooner you will want to change your life and eating habits.

Nutrition is a key part in the process of being healthy and living longer so get started today. The first step is the most important and the most significant.

INTRODUCTION

48 Sore Throat Juicing Solutions: Strengthen Your Immune System with These Life Changing Juice Recipes and Cure Your Sore Throat

By Joe Correa CSN

Each year about 13 million people in the USA alone suffer from a painful and dry feeling in the throat. This uncomfortable condition, sometimes followed by somewhat serious pain, is mostly caused by infections or some environmental factors like dry air or allergies. Luckily, the condition itself is not serious and will most likely go away on its own within a couple of days. If, however, you notice that the pain doesn't stop or is getting worse, visit your local doctor immediately.

There are several types of sore throat depending on the part of the throat that is affected.

-   Pharyngitis is an infection of the oral cavity (the area behind the mouth)
-   Tonsillitis affects the soft tissue in the back of the oral cavity known as tonsils
-   Laryngitis is the redness and/or swelling of the larynx (or the voice box)

The causes for this unpleasant condition can be divided into several categories:

- **Viral infections** cause about 90% of all sore throat conditions. These infections are related to common colds, flu, mononucleosis, and other virus-caused diseases
- **Bacterial Infections** are not as common as the viral infections and are mostly related to strep throat – an infection caused by Streptococcus bacteria
- **Allergies and dry air** are also a common cause of a sore throat condition. A body's reaction to some allergy triggers causes watery eyes, nasal congestion, sneezing, and sore throat. Dry air, on the other hand, soaks up the natural moisture from the mouth and throat causing the recognizable scratchy sensation.

Smoke and different chemicals are proven to irritate the throat and sometimes cause long-term infections and problems.

As someone who has been dealing with a sore throat for years, I have learned that the best way to prevent this irritating condition is to boost up the immune system and let the body defend itself.

This is why I wanted to share with you my favorite juice recipes that are proven to help fight off this condition and prevent them from happening in the future.

Make sure to try them all and see which ones suite you best.

COMMITMENT

In order to improve my condition, I *(your name)*, commit to eating more of these foods on a daily basis and to exercise at least 30 minutes daily:

- Berries (especially blueberries), peaches, cherries, apples, apricots, oranges, lemon juice, grapefruit, tangerines, mandarins, pears, etc.
- Broccoli, spinach, collard greens, sweet potatoes, avocado, artichoke, baby corn, carrots, celery, cauliflower, onions, etc.
- Whole grains, steel-cut oats, oatmeal, quinoa, barley, etc.
- Black beans, red bean beans, garbanzo beans, lentils, etc.
- Nuts and seeds including: walnuts, cashews, flaxseeds, sesame seeds, etc.
- Fish
- 8 – 10 glasses of water

Sign here

X_____

48 SORE THROAT JUICING SOLUTIONS

1.   Mango Lemon Juice

Ingredients:

1 cup mango, cubed

1 large lemon, peeled

1 cup sweet cherries, pitted

1 cup watermelon, cubed

1 tbsp liquid honey

2 oz water

Preparation:

Peel the mango and cut into small chunks. Set aside.

Peel the lemon and cut lengthwise in half. Set aside.

Wash the cherries under cold running water. Drain and cut in half. Remove the pits and set aside.

Cut the watermelon lengthwise. For one cup, you will need about 1 large wedge. Peel and cut into chunks.

Remove the seeds and set aside. Reserve the rest of the melon for some other juices.

Now, process mango, lemon, cherries, and watermelon in a juicer.

Transfer to serving glasses and add few ice cubes before serving.

Enjoy!

Nutrition information per serving: Kcal: 288, Protein: 4.6g, Carbs: 68.3g, Fats: 1.3g

2.   Carrot Melon Juice

Ingredients:

1 large carrot, sliced

1 large wedge of honeydew melon, peeled and cubed

1 cup cucumber, sliced

1 small ginger knob, 1-inch thick

1/8 tsp turmeric powder

2 oz water

Preparation:

Wash and peel the carrot. Cut into thin slices and set aside.

Cut melon lengthwise in half. Scoop out the seeds and then wash. Cut one large wedge and peel it. Cut into small cubes and set aside.

Wash the cucumber and cut into thin slices. Fill the measuring cup and reserve the rest for later. Set aside.

Peel the ginger knob and cut into small pieces. Set aside.

Now, combine carrot, melon, and cucumber in a juicer and process until juiced. Transfer to a serving glass and stir in the turmeric and water.

Refrigerate for 5 minutes before serving.

Nutrition information per serving: Kcal: 92, Protein: 2.6g, Carbs: 25.7g, Fats: 0.5g

3.   Agave Blueberry Juice

Ingredients:

2 cups fresh blueberries

1 cup black grapes

1 cup fresh mint, torn

1 large banana, peeled

1 tsp agave nectar

Preparation:

Place the blueberries in a colander. Rinse well under cold running water and drain. Set aside.

Wash the grapes and remove the stems. Fill the measuring cup and reserve the rest in the refrigerator. Set aside.

Wash the mint thoroughly under cold running water. Drain and torn into small pieces. Set aside.

Now, combine blueberries, grapes, mint, and banana in a juicer and process until juiced. Transfer to a serving glass and stir in the agave nectar.

Refrigerate for 5 minutes before serving.

Nutrition information per serving: Kcal: 326, Protein: 6.2g, Carbs: 93.4g, Fats: 2.1g

4.   Strawberry Ginger Juice

Ingredients:

1 cup fresh strawberries, chopped

1 small ginger knob, 1-inch thick

1 cup fresh kale, torn

1 whole lemon, peeled

Preparation:

Wash the strawberries under cold running water. Drain and set aside.

Peel the ginger knob and finely chop into tiny pieces. Set aside.

Place the kale in a colander and rinse thoroughly under cold running water. Drain and torn into small pieces. Set aside.

Peel the lemon and cut lengthwise in half. Set aside.

Combine strawberries, ginger, kale, and lemon in a juicer and process until juiced.

Transfer to serving glasses add some ice cubes before serving.

Enjoy!

Nutritional information per serving: Kcal: 120, Protein: 5.9g, Carbs: 38.6g, Fats: 1.8g

5.   Beet Apple Juice

Ingredients:

1 cup beet greens

1 medium-sized Granny Smith's apple, chopped

1 cup cantaloupe, diced

1 tbsp fresh mint, chopped

1 cup cauliflower, chopped

Preparation:

Wash the beet greens and torn with hands. Set aside.

Wash the apple and cut lengthwise in half. Remove the core and cut into bite-sized pieces. Set aside.

Cut the cantaloupe in half. Scoop out the seeds and flesh. Cut two wedges and peel them. Chop into chunks and set aside. Reserve the rest of the cantaloupe in a refrigerator.

Trim off the outer leaves of cauliflower. Wash it and cut into small pieces. Reserve the rest in the refrigerator.

Soak the mint leaves in hot water. Let it stand for 2 minutes.

Now, process beet greens, apple, cantaloupe, cauliflower,

and mint in a juicer.

Transfer to serving glasses and stir in the mint soaking water.

Refrigerate for 10-15 minutes before serving and enjoy.

Nutritional information per serving: Kcal: 123, Protein: 8.1g, Carbs: 37.7g, Fats: 1.1g

6. Grapefruit Orange Juice

Ingredients:

1 whole grapefruit, peeled

1 large orange, peeled

1 cup pineapple, chunked

1 cup cauliflower, chopped

¼ cup pure coconut water, unsweetened

Preparation:

Peel the grapefruit and orange and divide into wedges. Set aside.

Cut the top of a pineapple and peel it using a sharp knife. Cut into small chunks. Reserve the rest of the pineapple in a refrigerator.

Trim off the outer leaves of cauliflower. Wash it and cut into small pieces. Reserve the rest in the refrigerator.

Now, combine grapefruit, orange, pineapple, and cauliflower in a juicer and process until juiced. Transfer to serving glasses and stir in the pure coconut water.

Add few ice cubes and serve immediately.

Nutritional information per serving: Kcal: 247, Protein: 6.5g, Carbs: 74g, Fats: 1g

7.   Squash Nutmeg Juice

Ingredients:

1 cup butternut squash, chunked

1 cup avocado, chunked

½ tsp cinnamon, freshly ground

¼ tsp nutmeg, ground

¼ cup water

Preparation:

Peel the squash and cut in half. Scoop out the seeds using a spoon. Cut about 2 large wedges and pee. Cut the wedges into small chunks and fill the measuring cup. Reserve the rest in the refrigerator.

Peel and cut the avocado in half. Remove the pit and cut into small chunks. Set aside.

Now, combine squash and avocado in a juicer and process until juiced.

Transfer to serving glasses and stir in the water and cinnamon.

Serve immediately.

Nutritional information per serving: Kcal: 256, Protein: 5.3g, Carbs: 27.8g, Fats: 22.3g

8.   Blackberry Mint Juice

Ingredients:

1 cup blackberries

1 cup fresh mint, torn

1 cup cantaloupe, chopped

1 large orange, peeled

¼ tsp cinnamon, ground

Preparation:

Place the blackberries in a colander and rinse well. Drain and set aside.

Rinse the mint under cold running water and drain. Torn into small pieces and set aside.

Cut the cantaloupe in half. Scrape out the seeds and cut one large wedge. Peel and chop into small pieces. Fill the measuring cup and wrap the rest in a plastic foil. Refrigerate for later.

Peel the orange and divide into wedges. Cut each wedge in half and set aside.

Now, combine blackberries, mint, cantaloupe, and orange

in a juicer and process until juiced. Transfer to a serving glass and stir in the cinnamon. Optionally, add some water to increase the juice amount.

Serve immediately.

Nutrition information per serving: Kcal: 157, Protein: 5.9g, Carbs: 51.9g, Fats: 1.5g

9.   Cinnamon Pineapple Juice

Ingredients:

1 cup pineapple, chunked

1 whole lime, peeled and halved

1 small Granny Smith's apple, peeled and cored

1 tsp fresh mint leaves, finely chopped

¼ tsp cinnamon, ground

Preparation:

Cut the top of a pineapple and peel it using a sharp knife. Cut into small chunks and fill the measuring cup. Reserve the rest in the refrigerator.

Peel the lime and cut lengthwise in half. Set aside.

Wash the apple and remove the core. Cut into bite-sized pieces and set aside.

Process pineapple, lime, and apple in a juicer. Transfer to serving glasses and stir in the cinnamon. Add more water if needed.

Garnish with mint leaves and refrigerate before serving.

Nutritional information per serving: Kcal: 153, Protein: 1.7g, Carbs: 46.7g, Fats: 0.6g

10.   Mango Ginger Juice

Ingredients:

1 cup mango, chunked

1 small ginger slice

1 cup pomegranate seeds

1 medium-sized Gala apple, cored

1 oz coconut water

Preparation:

Peel the mango and cut into chunks. Fill the measuring cup and reserve the rest in the refrigerator. Set aside.

Peel the ginger slice and chop into small pieces. Set aside.

Cut the top of the pomegranate fruit using a sharp paring knife. Slice down to each of the white membranes inside of the fruit. Pop the seeds into a measuring cup and set aside.

Wash the apple and cut lengthwise in half. Remove the core and cut into small pieces. Set aside.

Now, combine mango, ginger, pomegranate seeds, and apple in a juicer and process until juiced. Transfer to a serving glass and stir in the cinnamon and water.

Refrigerate for 5 minutes before serving.

Nutrition information per serving: Kcal: 227, Protein: 3.6g, Carbs: 64.1g, Fats: 1.9g

11.   Orange Honey Juice

Ingredients:

3 large red oranges, peeled

1 tbsp honey, raw

1 large banana, peeled

1 tbsp fresh mint leaves, finely chopped

Preparation:

Peel the oranges and divide into wedges. Set aside.

Peel the banana and cut into small chunks. Set aside.

Process banana and oranges in a juicer. Transfer to serving glasses and stir in the honey.

Garnish with mint and refrigerate for 10 minutes before serving.

Enjoy!

Nutritional information per serving: Kcal: 123, Protein: 4.1g, Carbs: 73.9g, Fats: 1.1g

12. Mint Cucumber Juice

Ingredients:

1 large honeydew melon wedge, chopped

1 cup fresh mint, chopped

1 medium-sized cucumber, chopped

1 small Golden delicious apple, cored

1 oz coconut water

Preparation:

Place mint in a colander and wash thoroughly. Slightly drain and chop into small pieces. Set aside.

Wash the cucumber and cut into thin slices. Set aside.

Cut the melon in half. Cut one large wedge and peel the peel it. Cut into small pieces and set aside. Wrap the rest of the melon in a plastic foil and refrigerate for later.

Wash the apple and cut lengthwise in half. Remove the core and cut into bite-sized pieces. Set aside.

Now, combine mint, cucumber, melon, and apple in a juicer and process until juiced.

Transfer to a serving glass and stir in the water.

Optionally, add 1 tablespoon of lemon juice for a better taste. Refrigerate for 10 minutes before serving.

Enjoy!

Nutrition information per serving: Kcal: 139, Protein: 4.1g, Carbs: 40.5g, Fats: 0.9g

13.   Sour Cherry Juice

Ingredients:

2 cups sour cherries, pitted

1 medium-sized watermelon slice

1 cup celery, chopped

1 small ginger knob, peeled

1 oz water

Preparation:

Cut the watermelon in half. Cut one medium-sized wedge and wrap the rest in a plastic foil and refrigerate. Dice the wedge and remove the pits. Set aside.

Wash the celery and cut into small pieces. Fill the measuring cup and reserve the rest for later. Set aside.

Rinse the cherries under cold running water using a colander. Drain and cut each in half. Remove the pits and set aside.

Peel the ginger knob and cut into small pieces. Set aside.

Now, combine cherries, watermelon, celery, and ginger knob in a juicer and process until juiced. Transfer to a serving glass and stir in the water. Optionally, you can use coconut water if you like.

Serve immediately.

Nutrition information per serving: Kcal: 143, Protein: 3.4g, Carbs: 40.2g, Fats: 0.7g

14.   Sweet Berry Juice

Ingredients:

1 cup fresh cranberries

1 cup fresh blueberries

3 small Granny Smith's apples, cored

1 cup fresh kale, torn

1 tbsp liquid honey

Preparation:

Combine cranberries and blueberries in a colander and wash under cold running water. Drain and set aside.

Wash the apples and remove the core. Cut into bite-sized pieces and set aside.

Wash the kale thoroughly and torn with hands. Set aside.

Now, process cranberries, blueberries, apples, and kale in a juicer.

Transfer to serving glasses and stir in the honey. Add some ice or refrigerate before serving.

Nutrition information per serving: Kcal: 368, Protein: 5.6g, Carbs: 106g, Fats: 2.2g

15.   Cabbage Ginger Juice

Ingredients:

1 cup purple cabbage, chopped

1 small ginger knob, peeled and chopped

1 cup cauliflower, chopped

1 cup carrots, sliced

1 cup collard greens, chopped

Preparation:

Combine cabbage and collard greens in a colander. Wash thoroughly under cold running water and slightly drain. Chop into small pieces and set aside.

Peel the ginger knob and finely chop. Set aside.

Wash the cauliflower and trim off the outer leaves. Cut into bite-sized pieces and fill the measuring cup. Reserve the rest for later.

Wash and peel the carrots. Cut into thin slices and fill the measuring cup. Set aside.

Now, combine cabbage, ginger, cauliflower, carrots, and collard greens in a juicer and process until juiced. Transfer to a serving glass and refrigerate for 10 minutes before serving.

Nutrition information per serving: Kcal: 138, Protein: 5.3g, Carbs: 40.3g, Fats: 0.8g

16. Apple Carrot Juice

Ingredients:

2 large Gala apples, peeled and cored

3 medium-sized carrots, sliced

1 cup parsnips, sliced

¼ cup water

1 tbsp fresh lemon juice

Preparation:

Wash the apples and remove the core. Cut into bite-sized pieces and set aside.

Wash the carrots and parsnips and cut into thick slices. Set aside.

Now, combine apples, carrots, and parsnips in a juicer and process until juiced.

Transfer to serving glasses and stir in the water and lemon juice. Garnish with some mint and refrigerate before serving.

Enjoy!

Nutritional information per serving: Kcal: 332, Protein: 5.4g, Carbs: 100g, Fats: 1.6g

17.   Melon Blueberry Juice

Ingredients:

1 large wedge of honeydew melon

1 cup fresh blueberries

1 whole lemon, peeled and halved

1 large cucumber, sliced

Preparation:

Cut the honeydew melon lengthwise in half. Scoop out the seeds using a spoon. Cut the large wedges and peel them. Cut into small chunks and place in a bowl. Wrap the rest of the melon in a plastic foil and refrigerate.

Rinse the blueberries under cold running water. Drain and set aside.

Peel the lemon and cut lengthwise in half. Set aside.

Wash the cucumber and cut into thin slices. Set aside.

Now, process honeydew melon, blueberries, lemon, and cucumber in a juicer.

Transfer to serving glasses and add some ice if you like.

Serve immediately.

Nutritional information per serving: Kcal: 202, Protein: 5.5g, Carbs: 59.3g, Fats: 1.7g

18. Green Tomato Juice

Ingredients:

2 cups Iceberg lettuce, chopped

1 cup mustard greens, torn

1 cup parsley, torn

1 whole cucumber, sliced

1 large tomato, chopped

¼ tsp salt

Preparation:

Rinse the lettuce thoroughly under cold running water. Chop into small pieces and set aside.

Combine mustard greens and parsley in a large colander. Rinse well and drain. Torn into small pieces and set aside.

Wash the cucumber and cut into thin slices. Set aside.

Wash the tomato and place in a bowl. Chop into bite-sized pieces and reserve the tomato juice while cutting. Set aside.

Now, combine lettuce, mustard greens, parsley, cucumber, and tomato in a juicer and process until juiced.

Transfer to a serving glass and stir in the turmeric, salt, and reserved tomato juice.

Refrigerate for 5 minutes before serving.

Enjoy!

Nutrition information per serving: Kcal: 85, Protein: 7.6g, Carbs: 25.3g, Fats: 1.6g

19.　Sweet Orange Juice

Ingredients:

1 large orange, peeled

1 large peach, peeled

1 cup parsnip, sliced

1 tsp agave nectar

Preparation:

Wash the peach and cut in half. Remove the pit and cut into bite-sized pieces. Set aside.

Wash the parsnips and cut into thick slices. Set aside.

Peel the orange and divide into wedges. Set aside.

Now, process orange, peach, and parsnip in a juicer. Transfer to serving glasses and stir in the agave syrup.

Add some ice and serve immediately.

Nutritional information per serving: Kcal: 177, Protein: 5.2g, Carbs: 53.7g, Fats: 1.1g

20.   Carrot Kiwi Juice

Ingredients:

2 whole kiwis, peeled

1 cup carrots, chopped

2 cups green cabbage, shredded

1 whole grapefruit, peeled

1 tbsp honey, raw

Preparation:

Wash the carrots and cut into small pieces. Set aside.

Peel the kiwis and cut in half. Set aside.

Wash the cabbage thoroughly and roughly chop it using hands. Set aside.

Wash the grapefruit and cut into chunks. Set aside.

Now, process carrots, kiwis, cabbage, and grapefruit in a juicer. Transfer to a serving glass and stir in the honey.

Serve immediately.

Nutritional information per serving: Kcal: 219, Protein: 6.9g, Carbs: 69g, Fats: 1.5g

21. Apple Cantaloupe Juice

Ingredients:

1 small Red Delicious apple, cored

1 cup cantaloupe, cubed

1 cup fresh kale, torn

1 cup beets, sliced

¼ tsp ginger, ground

Preparation:

Wash the apple and cut lengthwise in half. Remove the core and cut into bite-sized pieces. Set aside.

Cut the cantaloupe in half. Scrape out the seeds and cut one large wedge. Peel and chop into small pieces. Fill the measuring cup and wrap the rest in a plastic foil. Refrigerate for later.

Rinse the kale thoroughly under cold running water. Drain and torn into small pieces. Set aside.

Wash the beets and trim off the green ends. Cut into thin slices and fill the measuring cup. Reserve the rest for some other juice.

Now, combine apple, cantaloupe, kale, and beets in a juicer and process until juiced. Transfer to a serving glass and stir in the ginger.

Add some ice and serve immediately.

Nutrition information per serving: Kcal: 181, Protein: 7g, Carbs: 51.1g, Fats: 1.4g

22.   Sweet Cucumber Melon Juice

Ingredients:

1 large cucumber, sliced

1 large honeydew melon wedge, chopped

1 cup watermelon, seeded

1 cup cantaloupe, cubed

1 tbsp liquid honey

Preparation:

Wash the cucumber and cut into thick slices. Set aside.

Cut the honeydew melon lengthwise in half. Scoop out the seeds using a spoon. Cut one large wedge and peel. Cut into small chunks and place in a bowl. Wrap the rest of the melon in a plastic foil and refrigerate.

Cut the watermelon lengthwise. For one cup, you will need about 1 large wedge. Peel and cut into chunks. Remove the seeds and set aside. Reserve the rest of for some other juices.

Cut the cantaloupe in half. Scoop out the seeds and flesh. Cut two wedges and peel them. Chop into chunks and set aside. Reserve the rest of the cantaloupe in a refrigerator.

Now, process cucumber, honeydew melon, watermelon, and cantaloupe in a juicer.

Transfer to serving glasses and stir in the honey.

Serve immediately and enjoy!

Nutritional information per serving: Kcal: 201, Protein: 3.4g, Carbs: 57.6g, Fats: 0.8g

23. Guava Lime Juice

Ingredients:

1 large guava, peeled

1 large lime, peeled

1 large cucumber

1 ripe avocado, pitted and peeled

2 oz coconut water

Preparation:

Peel the guava and cut into small chunks. Set aside.

Peel the lime and cut lengthwise in half. Set aside.

Wash the cucumber and cut into thick slices. Set aside.

Peel the avocado and cut in half. Remove the pit and cut into chunks. Set aside.

Now, process guava, lime, cucumber, and avocado in a juicer. Transfer to serving glasses and stir in the coconut water. Optionally, add some ginger if you like a bitter taste.

Add some ice and serve immediately.

Nutrition information per serving: Kcal: 352, Protein: 7.6g, Carbs: 41.6g, Fats: 30.3g

24.   Carrot Apple Juice

Ingredients:

1 large carrot, sliced

1 small Granny Smith's apple, cored and chopped

1 cup mango, chunked

1 medium-sized orange, wedged

1 oz coconut water

Preparation:

Wash and peel the carrot. Cut into bite-sized pieces and set aside.

Wash the apple and cut in half. Remove the core and cut into bite-sized pieces. Set aside.

Peel the mango and cut into chunks. Fill the measuring cup and reserve the rest for later.

Peel the orange and divide into wedges. Set aside.

Now, combine carrot, apple, mango, and orange in a juicer and process until juiced. Transfer to a serving glass and stir in the coconut water.

Serve immediately and enjoy!

Nutrition information per serving: Kcal: 189, Protein: 2.6g, Carbs: 56.4g, Fats:1.1g

25.   Sweet Coconut Juice

Ingredients:

½ cup pure coconut water, unsweetened

1 tsp agave nectar

1 Red Delicious apple, peeled and cored

1 medium-sized artichoke, chopped

1 cup fresh spinach, torn

½ tsp ginger, freshly ground

Preparation:

Wash the apple and remove the core. Cut into bite-sized pieces and set aside.

Using a sharp knife, trim off the outer leave of the artichoke. Cut into small pieces and set aside.

Rinse the spinach thoroughly under cold running water. Drain and torn into small pieces. Set aside.

Now, process apple, artichoke, and spinach in a juicer.

Transfer to serving glasses and stir in the ginger, coconut water, and agave nectar.

Add some ice and serve immediately.

Nutritional information per serving: Kcal: 195, Protein: 13.7g, Carbs: 63.4g, Fats: 1.3g

26.   Guava Lemon Juice

Ingredients:

1 whole guava, chopped

2 whole lemons, peeled

1 cup pineapple chunks

2 cups spinach, chopped

½ cup coconut water, unsweetened

Preparation:

Wash the guava and cut into chunks. If you are using large fruit, reserve the rest for some other recipe in a refrigerator.

Peel the lemons and cut lengthwise in half. Set aside.

Cut the top of a pineapple and peel it using a sharp knife. Cut into small chunks. Reserve the rest in the refrigerator.

Rinse the spinach thoroughly under cold running water. Torn with your hands and set aside.

Now, process guava, lemons, pineapple, and spinach and in a juicer. Transfer to serving glasses and stir in the coconut water.

Add some ice and serve immediately.

Nutritional information per serving: Kcal: 130, Protein: 4.8g, Carbs: 43g, Fats: 1.2g

27.   Beet Cauliflower Juice

Ingredients:

1 cup beets, trimmed

1 cup beet greens, chopped

1 cup cauliflower, chopped

1 cup parsnips, chopped

2 tbsp fresh mint, chopped

Preparation:

Wash the beets and trim off the green parts. Cut into small pieces. Chop the greens and set aside.

Trim off the outer leaves of a cauliflower. Wash it and chop into small pieces. Set aside.

Rinse the parsnips and cut into thick slices. Set aside.

Now, process beets, beet greens, cauliflower, and parsnips in a juicer.Transfer to serving glasses and garnish with some fresh mint before serving.

Enjoy!

Nutritional information per serving: Kcal: 166, Protein: 9.9g, Carbs: 52.3g, Fats: 1.5g

28.   Pineapple Mint Juice

Ingredients:

1 cup pineapple, chunked

1 cup fresh mint, torn

1 cup cucumber, sliced

1 whole guava, chopped

1 oz coconut water

Preparation:

Cut the top of the pineapple and peel it using a sharp paring knife. Peel it and cut into small pieces. Fill the measuring cup and reserve the rest in the refrigerator. Set aside.

Wash the mint and slightly drain. Torn with hands and set aside.

Wash the cucumber and cut into thin slices. Fill the measuring cup and reserve the rest in the refrigerator.

Wash and peel the guava fruit. Chop into bite-sized pieces and set aside.

Now, combine pineapple, mint, cucumber, and guava in a

juicer and process until juiced. Transfer to a serving glass and stir in the water.

Refrigerate for 5 minutes before serving.

Nutrition information per serving: Kcal: 115, Protein: 3.6g, Carbs: 35.2g, Fats: 1.1g

29.   Avocado Lime Juice

Ingredients:

1 cup avocado, peeled and pitted

1 large lime, peeled

2 large honeydew melon wedges

5 tbsp fresh mint

1 medium-sized pineapple slice, chopped

Preparation:

Peel the avocado and cut in half. Remove the pit and cut into chunks. Add it to the bowl with melon and set aside.

Peel the lime and cut lengthwise in half. Set aside.

Cut the honeydew melon lengthwise in half. Scoop out the seeds using a spoon. Cut the large wedges and peel them. Cut into small chunks and place in a bowl. Wrap the rest of the melon in a plastic foil and refrigerate.

Wash the mint leaves and soak in water for 5 minutes.

Now, process avocado, lime, honeydew melon, mint, and pineapple in a juicer. Transfer to serving glasses and serve immediately.

Enjoy!

Nutritional information per serving: Kcal: 321, Protein: 5.2g, Carbs: 46.8g, Fats: 22.6g

30.   Spinach Apple Juice

Ingredients:

½ cup spinach, torn

1 large Gala apple, cored

½ tsp ginger, ground

1 large cucumber

¼ cup fresh parsley, finely chopped

Preparation:

Rinse the spinach and parsley using a large colander. Drain and chop into small pieces. Set aside.

Core the apple and chop into bite-sized pieces. Place it in a medium bowl and set aside.

Chop the cucumber into thick slices and combine it with an apple.

Roughly chop the parsley and collard greens and combine it with remaining prepared ingredients.

Process all in a juicer until well juiced. Transfer to serving glasses and stir in the ginger.

Add some ice cubes or refrigerate before serving.

Enjoy!

Nutritional information per serving: Kcal: 96, Protein: 3.1g, Carbs: 28.7g, Fats: 1.2g

31.   Salted Tomato Asparagus Juice

Ingredients:

3 large tomatoes, chopped

1 cup asparagus, trimmed and chopped

4 large carrots,sliced

2 medium-sized zucchinis, peeled and chopped

¼ tsp salt

Preparation:

Wash the tomatoes and cut into quarters. Cut in a bowl to reserve the juices. Set aside.

Wash the carrots and cut into small pieces. Set aside.

Peel the zucchinis and remove the seeds. Cut into bite-sized chunks and set aside.

Wash the asparagus and remove the woody ends. Chop into small pieces and set aside.

Combine tomatoes, carrots, zucchinis, and asparagus in a juicer and process until juiced.

Transfer to serving glasses and add a little bit of milk to adjust the thickness of the juice. Stir in the salt.

Serve immediately.

Nutrition information per serving: Kcal: 92, Protein: 5.4g, Carbs: 27.3g, Fats: 0.9g

32.   Ginger Pomegranate Juice

Ingredients:

1 tsp fresh ginger, freshly grated

½ cup pomegranate seeds

½ cup fresh kale, torn

1 large Granny Smith's apple, cored

1 tbsp agave nectar

Preparation:

Peel the ginger knob and grate. Fill up the measuring teaspoon and reserve the rest in the refrigerator.

Cut the top of the pomegranate fruit using a sharp knife. slice down to each of the white membranes inside of the fruit. Pop the seeds into a medium sized bowl.

Rinse the kale thoroughly. Drain and torn into small pieces. Set aside.

Wash the apple and remove the core. Cut into bite-sized pieces and set aside.

Process the pomegranate seeds, kale, and apple in a juicer until well juiced.

Transfer to serving glasses and stir in the ginger. Add some water to adjust the thickness and stir in the agave nectar.

Serve immediately.

Nutrition information per serving: Kcal: 194, Protein: 6.2g, Carbs: 54.2g, Fats: 2.4g

33.   Lemon Chia Juice

Ingredients:

1 whole lemon, peeled

3 tbsp chia seeds

1 large yellow bell pepper, seeded

1 large Red Delicious apple, cored

Preparation:

Peel the lemon and cut into quarters. Set aside.

Wash the bell pepper and cut into halves. Remove the seeds and chop into small pieces.

Wash the apple and remove the core. Cut into bite-sized pieces and set aside.

Combine bell pepper, apple, and lemon in a juicer. Process until juiced.

Transfer to serving glasses and stir in the chia seeds. Add 2-3 tablespoons of water and stir again.

Stir well and serve immediately..

Enjoy!

Nutrition information per serving: Kcal: 135, Protein: 4.2g, Carbs: 31.3g, Fats: 6.2g

34.   Artichoke Spinach Juice

Ingredients:

1 cup artichoke, chopped

1 cup fresh spinach, torn

1 cup avocado, cubed

1 cup green cabbage, torn

¼ tsp ginger powder

Preparation:

Trim off the outer layers of the artichoke using a sharp paring knife. Cut into bite-sized pieces and fill the measuring cup. Reserve the rest for later.

Combine spinach and cabbage in a large colander. Wash thoroughly under cold running water. Drain and torn into small pieces. Set aside.

Peel the avocado and cut lengthwise in half. Remove the pit and cut into small cubes. Fill the measuring cup and reserve the rest in the refrigerator.

Now, combine artichoke, spinach, avocado, and cabbage in a juicer and process until juiced. Transfer to a serving glass and stir in the ginger powder.

Refrigerate for 10 minutes before serving.

Nutrition information per serving: Kcal: 282, Protein: 15.4g, Carbs: 42.6g, Fats: 23.2g

35. Lemon Mango Juice

Ingredients:

2 whole lemons, peeled and halved

1 cup mango, chunked

1 whole grapefruit, peeled and wedged

1 small Red Delicious apple, cored

¼ tsp ginger, ground

1 tbsp agave nectar

Preparation:

Peel the lemons and cut each lengthwise in half. Set aside.

Peel the mango and cut into chunks. Fill the measuring cup and reserve the rest for later. Set aside.

Peel the grapefruit and divide into wedges. Cut each wedge in half and set aside.

Wash the apple and cut lengthwise in half. Remove the core and cut into bite-sized pieces. Set aside.

Now, combine lemon, mango, grapefruit, and apple in a juicer and process until juiced. Transfer to serving glasses and stir in the ginger, milk, and agave.

Add few ice cubes and serve immediately.

Enjoy!

Nutrition information per serving: Kcal: 155, Protein: 4.5g, Carbs: 23.8g, Fats: 1.8g

36.   Ginger Plum Juice

Ingredients:

1 whole plum, chopped

¼ tsp ginger, ground

1 cup cantaloupe, chopped

1 cup fresh mint, torn

1 large orange, peeled

Preparation:

Cut the cantaloupe in half. Scoop out the seeds and flesh. Cut and peel one large wedge. Chop into chunks and fill the measuring cup. Reserve the rest of the cantaloupe in a refrigerator.

Wash the mint thoroughly under cold running water. Torn into small pieces and set aside.

Peel the orange and divide into wedges. Cut each wedge in half and set aside.

Wash the plum and cut in half. Remove the pit and chop into small pieces. Set aside.

Now, combine plum, cantaloupe, mint, and orange in a

juicer and process until juiced. Transfer to a serving glass and stir in the ginger.

Serve immediately.

Nutrition information per serving: Kcal: 151, Protein: 4.4g, Carbs: 45.6g, Fats: 0.9g

37. Sour Fuji Cinnamon Juice

Ingredients:

1 large Fuji apple, cored

1 whole lime, peeled

¼ tsp cinnamon, ground

1 cup watermelon, chopped

1 large banana, chopped

1 cup fresh mint, torn

Preparation:

Wash the apple and cut lengthwise in half. Remove the core and chop into bite-sized pieces. Set aside.

Peel the lime and cut lengthwise in half. Set aside.

Wash the mint thoroughly under cold running water. Drain and torn into small pieces. Set aside.

Cut the watermelon in half. Cut one large wedge and wrap the rest in a plastic foil and refrigerate. Peel the slice and cut into small cubes. Remove the pits and fill the measuring cup. Set aside.

Peel the banana and cut into small chunks. Set asid

Now, combine apple, lime, watermelon, banana, and mint in a juicer and process until juiced. Transfer to a serving glass and stir in the cinnamon.

Add some crushed ice and serve immediately.

Nutrition information per serving: Kcal: 236, Protein: 4.6g, Carbs: 66.4g, Fats: 1.1g

38. Lemon Honey Juice

Ingredients:

1 whole lemon, peeled

1 tsp liquid honey

1 cup grapefruit, chopped

2 large oranges, peeled

¼ tsp of ginger, ground

Preparation:

Peel the lemon and cut into quarters. Set aside.

Peel the grapefruit and divide into wedges.. Cut each wedge in half and set aside.

Peel the oranges and divide into wedges. Set aside.

Wash the kale leaves and roughly chop it.

Now, process lemon,grapefruit, and oranges in a juicer. Transfer to serving glasses and add some water to adjust the thickness if needed. Stir in the liquid honey and ginger.

Serve immediately.

Nutrition information per serving: Kcal: 128, Protein: 7.3g, Carbs: 34.5g, Fats: 1.1g

39.   Orange Cinnamon Juice

Ingredients:

1 large orange, peeled

2 large carrots, sliced

1 cup fresh strawberries

2 large Granny Smith's apples, cored

¼ tsp cinnamon, ground

Preparation:

Peel the orange and divide into wedges. Set aside.

Wash carrots and cut into small pieces. Set aside.

Wash strawberries and cut them into halves. Set aside.

Wash apples and cut in half. Remove the core and cut into bite-sized pieces. Set aside.

Now, process orange, carrots, strawberries, and apples in a juicer. Transfer to the serving glasses and stir in the cinnamon. Optionally, add some water if needed.

Refrigerate for 15 minutes before serving.

Nutrition information per serving: Kcal: 104, Protein:

3.9g, Carbs: 31.2g, Fats: 1.1g

40. Pomegranate Lime Juice

Ingredients:

1 cup pomegranate seeds

1 whole lime, peeled

1 small Granny Smith's apple, cored

1 cup blueberries

¼ tsp ginger, ground

2 oz water

Preparation:

Cut the top of the pomegranate fruit using a sharp paring knife. Slice down to each of the white membranes inside of the fruit. Pop the seeds into a measuring cup and set aside.

Peel the lime and cut lengthwise in half. Set aside.

Wash the apple and cut lengthwise in half. Remove the core and cut into bite-sized pieces and set aside.

Place the blueberries in a colander. Rinse well under cold running water and drain. Set aside.

Now, combine pomegranate seeds, lime, apple, and

blueberries in a juicer and process until juiced. Transfer to a serving glass and stir in the ginger and water.

Refrigerate for 5 minutes before serving.

Enjoy!

Nutrition information per serving: Kcal: 206, Protein: 3.3g, Carbs: 61.1g, Fats: 1.8g

41.   Ginger Banana Juice

Ingredients:

1 banana, sliced

¼ tsp ginger powder

1 large celery stalk, chopped

1 small Granny Smith' apple, cored

1 tbsp aloe juice

1 cup cucumber, sliced

Preparation:

Peel the banana and cut into chunks. Set aside.

Wash the celery stalk and chop into bite-sized pieces. Set aside.

Wash the apple and cut in half. Remove the core and cut into bite-sized pieces. Set aside.

Wash the cucumber and cut into thin slices. Fill the measuring cup and reserve the rest for later. Set aside.

Now, combine banana, celery apple, and cucumber in a juicer. Process until juiced.

Transfer to a serving glass and stir in the aloe juice and ginger. Optionally, stir in some fresh lemon juice for a bitter taste.

Add some crushed ice and serve immediately.

Nutrition information per serving: Kcal: 174, Protein: 2.7g, Carbs: 50.3g, Fats: 0.8g

42.   Cucumber Zucchini Juice

Ingredients:

1 cup cucumber, sliced

1 small zucchini, chopped

1 cup watercress, chopped

1 cup parsnip, sliced

¼ tsp ginger, ground

1 oz water

Preparation:

Wash the watercress thoroughly under cold running water. Drain and chop into small pieces. Set aside.

Wash the cucumber and cut into thin slices. Fill the measuring cup and reserve the rest for later. Set aside.

Peel the zucchini and cut into thin slices. Set aside.

Wash the parsnip and trim off the green parts. slightly peel and cut into slices. Set side.

Now, combine watercress, cucumber, zucchini, and parsnip in a juicer and process until juiced. Transfer to a serving glass and stir in the water and ginger.

Add some ice and serve immediately.

Nutrition information per serving: Kcal: 100, Protein: 4.2g, Carbs: 29.9g, Fats: 0.9g

43.   Apple Ginger Juice

Ingredients:

1 small Golden Delicious apple, cored

1 small ginger knob, peeled and sliced

1 small pear, cored and chopped

1 medium-sized banana, peeled and chunked

1 cup fresh spinach, chopped

Preparation:

Wash the apple and cut in half. Remove the core and cut into bite-sized pieces. Set aside.

Peel the ginger knob and chop into small pieces. Set aside.

Wash the pear and remove the core. Cut into small pieces and set aside.

Peel the banana and cut into small chunks. Set aside.

Wash the spinach thoroughly under cold running water. Slightly drain and chop into small pieces. Set aside.

Now, combine apple, ginger, pear, banana, and spinach in a juicer and process until juiced. Transfer to a serving glass and refrigerate for 10-15 minutes before serving.

Enjoy!

Nutrition information per serving: Kcal: 247, Protein: 1.7g, Carbs: 73.9g, Fats: 1.7g

44. Cantaloupe Mint Juice

Ingredients:

1 small Red Delicious apple, cored

1 large wedge of cantaloupe, chopped

1 cup fresh mint, chopped

1 cup mustard greens, chopped

1 oz milk

Preparation:

Cut the cantaloupe in half. Cut one large wedge and peel it. Cut into small pieces and set aside. Wrap the rest of the melon in a plastic foil and refrigerate for later.

Combine mint and mustard greens in a colander and wash thoroughly. Slightly drain and chop into small pieces. Set aside.

Wash the apple and cut lengthwise in half. Remove the core and cut into bite-sized pieces. Set aside.

Now, combine cantaloupe, mint, apple, and mustard greens in a juicer and process until juiced.

Transfer to a serving glass and stir in the water.

Refrigerate for 10 minutes before serving.

Nutrition information per serving: Kcal: 152, Protein: 5.6g, Carbs: 41.7g, Fats: 1.3g

45.   Orange Broccoli Juice

Ingredients:

1 large orange, peeled

1 cup broccoli, chopped

2 oz coconut water

1 whole lime, peeled and halved

1 cup cucumber, sliced

¼ tsp ginger, ground

Preparation:

Peel the orange and divide into wedges. Cut each wedge in half and set aside.

Wash the broccoli and trim off the outer leaves. Cut into small pieces and fill the measuring cup. Reserve the rest in the refrigerator.

Peel the lime and cut lengthwise in half. Set aside.

Wash the cucumber and cut into thin slices. Fill the measuring cup and reserve the rest for later.

Now, combine orange, broccoli, lime, and cucumber in a juicer and process until juiced. Transfer to a serving glass and stir in the coconut water and ginger. Add some ice and serve immediately.

Nutrition information per serving: Kcal: 106, Protein: 4.8g, Carbs: 33.3g, Fats: 0.6g

46.   Green Vegetable Juice

Ingredients:

1 cup collard greens, torn

¼ tsp ginger, ground

1 tsp green tea powder

2 cups spinach, torn

1 cup watercress, torn

1 cup kale, torn

1 oz water

Preparation:

Combine collard greens spinach, watercress, and kale in a large colander. Wash thoroughly under cold running water. Slightly drain and torn into small pieces.

Place the tea powder in a small bowl. Add 3 tbsp of hot water and stir well. Set aside for 3 minutes.

Now, combine Swiss chard, spinach, watercress, and kale in a juicer and process until juiced. Transfer to a serving glass and stir in the ginger and water.

Refrigerate for 10 minutes before serving.

Enjoy!

Nutrition information per serving: Kcal: 87, Protein: 16.3g, Carbs: 22.9g, Fats: 2.4g

47.   Tropical Grapefruit Ginger Juice

Ingredients:

1 whole grapefruit, peeled

¼ tsp ginger, ground

1 cup papaya, chopped

1 large orange, peeled

1 cup cucumber, sliced

2 tbsp coconut water

Preparation:

Peel the papaya and cut into small chunks. Fill the measuring cup and reserve the rest in the refrigerator.

Peel the grapefruit and orange. Divide into wedges. Cut each wedge in half and set aside.

Wash the cucumber and cut into thin slices. Fill the measuring cup and reserve the rest for later.

Now, combine grapefruit, papaya, orange, and cucumber in a juicer and process until well juiced.

Transfer to a serving glass and stir in the ginger and coconut water.

Refrigerate for 10 minutes before serving.

Nutrition information per serving: Kcal: 214, Protein: 4.6g, Carbs: 65.4g, Fats: 1g

48.   Strawberry Mint Juice

Ingredients:

1 cup strawberries, chopped

1 cup fresh mint, torn

1 small Golden Delicious apple, core and chopped

¼ tsp cinnamon, ground

1 cup honeydew melon, diced

Preparation:

Wash the strawberries and remove the stems. Cut into bite-sized pieces and set aside.

Rinse the mint thoroughly and slightly drain. Torn with hands and set aside.

Wash the apple and cut in half. Remove the core and cut into bite-sized pieces. Set aside.

Cut the top of the melon. Cut lengthwise in half and then cut one large wedge. Peel the wedge and cut into small cubes. Remove the seeds and fill the measuring cup. Wrap the rest in a plastic foil and refrigerate.

Now, combine strawberries, mint, apple and honeydew

melon in a juicer and process until juiced. Transfer to a serving glass and stir in the cinnamon.

Add some crushed ice and serve immediately.

Nutrition information per serving: Kcal: 153, Protein: 3.5g, Carbs: 43.3g, Fats: 1.1g

ADDITIONAL TITLES FROM THIS AUTHOR

70 Effective Meal Recipes to Prevent and Solve Being Overweight: Burn Fat Fast by Using Proper Dieting and Smart Nutrition

By Joe Correa CSN

48 Acne Solving Meal Recipes: The Fast and Natural Path to Fixing Your Acne Problems in Less Than 10 Days!

By Joe Correa CSN

41 Alzheimer's Preventing Meal Recipes: Reduce or Eliminate Your Alzheimer's Condition in 30 Days or Less!

By Joe Correa CSN

70 Effective Breast Cancer Meal Recipes: Prevent and Fight Breast Cancer with Smart Nutrition and Powerful Foods

By Joe Correa CSN

9 781635 318043